How to Prevent and Possibly Reverse the Effects of Dementia

By Shawn Konecni, PhD

Printed in the United States of America

First Printing, 2016

ISBN-13: 978-0-9913191-2-1

Breakout Concepts LLC

Contact – bcinfo@breakoutconcepts.com

Disclaimer

The information presented in this book is intended for informational and educational purposes only. The author and publisher have made every effort to ensure that the information contained herein is as accurate as possible at the time of writing. It cannot contain all of the information available on any one subject and some of the information may not be up-to-date. As such, the information is provided on an as-is basis. Any errors or omissions, whether typographical or in content, are unintentional.

Furthermore, this book should not be used as a substitute for professional medical advice. You should not use this information to diagnose or treat any medical condition. Consult your healthcare provider before starting any diet or exercise program, before taking any medication, or if you suspect you have any health problem. Any use or misuse of the information contained in this book is solely the responsibility of the user.

Table of Contents

What is Dementia

Dementia is defined as a decline in mental ability, caused by damage to brain cells [1]. It is a chronic condition, and it is often progressive. The exact nature of the condition varies depending on the type of dementia and the overall health of the individual. However, there are some common signs. For example, a person suffering from dementia may become more forgetful and lose his or her keys more often than usual. The same person may get lost when leaving the house, and may have trouble making decisions or planning events. Or, he or she may have difficulty following conversations or may have trouble coming up with the right words to express an idea. Such changes in mental ability and behavior are synonymous with the more common forms of dementia. Obviously, all of these changes can have a significant effect on one's quality of life.

Dementia is not, in and of itself, a disease. It is a condition, or disorder, that comes with certain symptoms. Contrary to popular belief, it is not a natural byproduct of aging, although the risk of developing dementia increases as one grows older.

There are various types of dementia. The most common type is called Alzheimer's disease. Alzheimer's disease is a well-known chronic disease, and is one of the leading causes of death in the United States [2]. Another type of dementia is related to stroke, which is also a leading cause of death. As such, dementia is a condition that adversely affects a large number of people.

There is, unfortunately, no known cure for most types of dementia, including Alzheimer's disease. There are a handful of treatments, but these only mitigate, or relieve, symptoms. Despite having few options, we do not have to give up and wait for the condition to develop. The biggest weapon we have against dementia is prevention and common sense. We can and should do everything within our means to decrease the risk of developing dementia in the first place.

However, what if we develop dementia due to factors outside of our control? The good news is that we do not simply have to accept this condition with no recourse. If we are beyond the prevention stage, we can still take action on our own to possibly reverse the effects, even after we begin to exhibit symptoms. Naturally, if dementia has progressed beyond the early stages, such a feat becomes vastly more difficult. Still, we have to keep fighting.

Of course, none of what is described here is meant to replace modern medicine, or the treatments that are prescribed or recommended by a doctor or healthcare provider. At the same time, we do not have to accept that this is all there is to help us. We can, and should, take responsibility for our own health. We can improve the odds to avoid dementia altogether. And even if we can't avoid dementia, we may still have the ability to slow down this condition so we can maintain our quality-of-life to some extent.

Why you need this Book

Whether dementia runs in your family or you know someone who has it, you are probably concerned about the prospect of a dementia diagnosis. You may have observed some mental decline or suspicious behavior in people who are close to you, or you may have experienced a few early symptoms yourself. Regardless of the reason, this book is here to help.

Consider this book as a primer on dementia. It is meant to be a tool to help sift through an abundance of complex information to reveal what you can do to reduce risk and mitigate symptoms. It is not meant to be a definitive guide or a textbook. There are plenty of detailed resources on the Internet for that and many of them are free. The purpose of this book is to help you, the reader, understand the problems that dementia poses. It is intended to enable you, or someone close to you, to move quickly towards a simple goal – to live a healthy life without dementia or without having to suffer from the symptoms of dementia. Such information is even more important as you age.

It is possible to be proactive and reduce the risk of developing dementia. When it comes to Alzheimer's disease, for example, research has suggested that approximately one out of three cases is preventable [3]. This is just for one type of dementia and is based on limited data. You can be part of this statistic. To reduce risk, this book will explain how to **eliminate triggers that lead to dementia**. Examples of such triggers include poor nutrition, unhealthy habits, or associated chronic diseases that have been linked to dementia.

In the event that dementia is not preventable, you should do everything in your capacity to delay the onset of symptoms, for as long as possible. This book will suggest a variety of ways to reinforce and heal the brain. In a nutshell, you need to **engage in mental and physical activities that make the brain more resilient to dementia**.

No matter how you approach this problem, preventive measures are more effective if applied early, so there is no time to waste. Let's get started by learning more about dementia.

What Happens to the Brain

When we age, our brain starts to shrink and blood circulation is reduced. Brain cells (also called neurons) begin to degrade. Structures, called plaques and tangles, may begin to form. Such changes can cause damage to brain cells, or at the very least, cause them to malfunction [4]. This damage occurs rather slowly and is responsible for the observed mental decline in some people as they age.

Dementia, on the other hand, is caused by accelerated, and sometimes widespread, damage to brain cells. These brain cells, which were once healthy, stop functioning properly. Eventually the malfunctioning cells are lost for good. Even though there are numerous neurons in the brain (billions), the continued loss of neurons over time begins to take its toll.

Communication between brain cells occurs over trillions of physical connections. The connections form over the course of one's life and change based on one's experiences and interactions with the environment. They are a network of conduits, in a sense, for communication, and with the loss of brain cells, some of the connections are similarly lost. Without these connections, we cannot think properly. As the brain cell count decreases and connections are lost, mental abilities, personality, and feelings are affected. We begin to notice more and more symptoms over time.

Depending on the type of dementia, damage can be focused in a particular region of the brain. Each region of the brain handles different critical functions, such as memory, decision-making, vision, speech, and muscle control. When neurons and their connections are damaged in a certain region, the associated functionality is compromised. In other words, normal brain function may no longer be possible.

Damage can also be more distributed across the brain, affecting multiple regions simultaneously. For example, in the most common form of dementia, Alzheimer's disease, damage is very widespread and many brain cells are lost, in turn losing their connections to other cells. The result is a more serious loss of functionality and, after a certain amount of time, is fatal.

Types of Dementia

There are multiple types of dementia, and a person exhibiting signs of dementia may be suffering from one or more types. Experiencing more than one type of dementia is commonly referred to as **mixed dementia**. For more common individual types of dementia, the following gives a brief overview of each one [5].

• **Alzheimer's disease** – This is the most common type of dementia. It comprises an estimated two out of three of all dementia cases. Alzheimer's is a progressive disease that results in widespread damage. The exact cause is unknown, but it is accompanied by the buildup of protein deposits (called plaques) and twisted protein strands (called tangles) in the brain. The protein buildup appears to disrupt brain cell function and may be responsible for brain cell loss. Common symptoms include problems with memory, thinking, and behavior.

• **Vascular dementia** – This is the second most common type of dementia. It is caused by lack of blood flow in the brain. Without adequate blood flow, the brain cannot receive oxygen and nutrients needed to function. Vascular dementia usually follows a stroke, but can be attributed to other conditions as well [6]. Symptoms of vascular dementia are varied and will be largely dependent upon the location and extent of the damage to the brain.

• **Dementia with Lewy bodies (DLB)** – This dementia is associated with the buildup of protein deposits (called Lewy bodies) in the brain. Like Alzheimer's disease, this buildup appears to disrupt brain cell function and may be responsible for brain cell loss. It is the third most common type of dementia and sometimes accompanies other dementias, including Alzheimer's disease and vascular dementia. Symptoms are similar to that of Alzheimer's, but can include sleep problems, hallucinations, and problems with movement.

• **Parkinson's disease** – This type of dementia is similar to DLB. Common symptoms include problems with movement.

• **Frontotemporal dementia** – This type of dementia affects multiple areas of the brain, including the frontal and temporal lobes. The exact cause is unknown. Common symptoms include changes in personality and behavior, and problems with language.

• **Creutzfeldt-Jakob disease (CJD)** – This form of dementia is rare and is caused by abnormal proteins (known as prions) that form in the brain. Common symptoms include memory and thinking problems, loss of coordination, changes in behavior, and problems with movement. CJD is marked by its rapid progression and brain deterioration, and symptoms get worse very quickly.

• **Huntington's disease** – This type of dementia is caused by a genetic disorder. The most common symptoms are involuntary movements, changes in personality and behavior, and problems with thinking and reasoning.

• **Wernicke-Korsakoff Syndrome** – This form of dementia is considered to be preventable. It is caused by a severe vitamin B1 deficiency (Thiamine) due to excessive alcohol consumption. Common symptoms include memory problems.

Regions of the Brain and Loss of Function

Some dementias, such as Alzheimer's disease, affect the entire brain, while others, such as vascular dementia and frontotemporal dementia, are known to affect specific areas. As dementia progresses, certain areas of the brain may be more affected than others.

Damage to any specific region of the brain can result in loss of function, resulting in observed symptoms. To briefly elaborate on brain function, the following is a breakdown of the four main regions of the brain, also known as brain lobes [7, 8].

• **Frontal lobe** – This region of the brain is located near the forehead. Functions include personality, behavior, emotions, judgement, planning, problem solving, speech, movement, intelligence, concentration, and self-awareness. Damage in this region can result in changes in personality and behavior, problems with speech and expression of ideas, difficulty processing new information, delayed responses to questions, difficulty with problem solving, lack of interest, weakness, and paralysis.

Frontal Lobe

- *Personality, behavior, emotions*
- *Judgement, planning, problem solving*
- *Speaking, writing*
- *Voluntary body movement*
- *Intelligence, concentration, self-awareness*

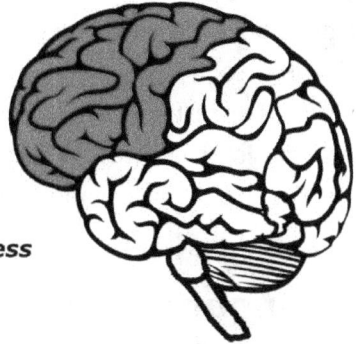

*   *   *

• **Parietal lobe** – This region is located near the back and top of the head. Functions include interpretation of language and words, sense of touch, integration of sensory input, and spatial and visual perception. Damage in this region can result in numbness or lack of touch sensation (e.g. can't feel pain, heat, cold, and vibration), difficulty recognizing objects by touch (e.g. can't recognize texture and shape), disorientation, confusion, difficulty with writing and doing calculations, and difficulty performing simple tasks such as getting dressed or doing basic chores. It may also result in difficulty recognizing how objects relate to each other in space, which leads to problems with tasks such as drawing or putting things together.

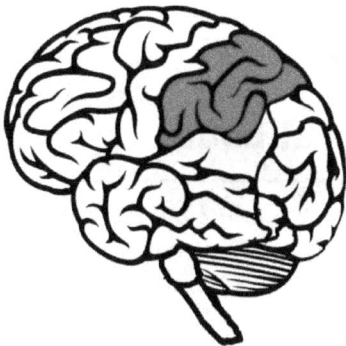

Parietal Lobe

- *Interpretation of langauge, words*
- *Sense of touch, pain, temperature*
- *Integration of signals from vision, hearing, movement, touch, memory*
- *Spatial, visual perception, navigation*

• **Temporal lobe** – This region is located at the side of the head, on both sides, above the ears. Functions include language comprehension, memory, hearing, sequencing, and organization of information. Damage in this region can result in loss of memory (e.g. can't remember words, sounds, and music), problems with language comprehension, the inability to think clearly, and changes in mood and personality.

Temporal Lobe

• *Language comprehension*
• *Memory*
• *Hearing*
• *Sequencing of actions*
• *Organization of information*

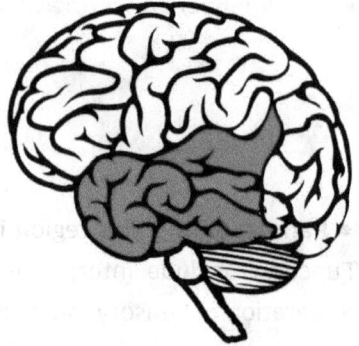

*   *   *

• **Occipital lobe** – This region is located near the back of the head. Functions include interpretation of visual information including, color, light, and movement. Damage in this region can result in loss of eyesight, problems recognizing familiar objects and faces, problems interpreting what is seen, and hallucinations.

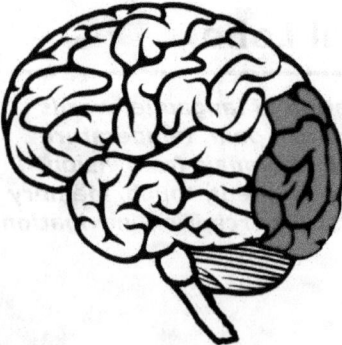

Occipital Lobe

• *Interpretation of visual information*
• *Interpretation of color, light, movement*

Note that there is some overlap between the regions when it comes to function and this overlap is more pronounced when doing complex tasks. For example, doing mathematical calculations would require both the frontal and parietal lobes. Having a verbal conversation would require the frontal, parietal, and temporal lobes.

Common Signs of Dementia

Diagnosing any type of dementia without the help of a medical professional is largely subjective, especially in the early stages. Every person is different, and signs (or symptoms) can vary depending on the specific brain disease and whether the damage is localized or widespread. However, taking note of some of the signs could give an early warning.

As mentioned earlier, dementia is often progressive, which means symptoms start out slowly and gradually get worse over time. Of course, any noticeable progressive condition is an obvious sign that something might be wrong. After all, we can all be forgetful from time to time, but, this alone does not mean that we have dementia. It is expected that we may slow down a bit as we get older [4]. For example, it may take longer to perform certain complex tasks or we may have a harder time learning new things. This does not mean we have dementia. If we take a little more time to perform a task, but we can still get the job done, we can probably attribute such performance issues to the aging process. If, however, we encounter symptoms that are unusual, occur repeatedly, or get progressively worse in a short amount of time, further evaluation may be warranted.

To get an idea of what progressive symptoms of dementia might look like, the following are common signs observed at the early, middle, and later stages [9, 10].

Early-stage signs:

• Shows signs of forgetfulness more often

• Shows unusually-poor judgement more often

• Misplaces items (e.g. keys, cellphones, dentures, and jewelry)

• Loses track of time

• Becomes lost in familiar places (e.g. gets lost on own street, forgets how to get home)

Middle-stage signs:

• Experiences recent memory loss (e.g. forgets recent events or people's names)

• Becomes lost at home

• Has increased difficulty with communication (e.g. forgets simple words or uses the wrong words)

• Needs help with personal care

• Experiences behavioral changes (e.g. becomes irritable or suspicious more often)

• Repeats the same questions over and over

• Exhibits wandering tendencies, which can result in getting lost more often

Late-stage signs:

• Becomes unaware of time and place

• Has difficulty recognizing relatives and friends

- Has an increasing need for assistance with personal care

- Has difficulty walking

- Experiences escalated behavioral changes (e.g. becomes increasingly aggressive)

*   *   *

At an early stage, it is not uncommon to overlook symptoms of dementia. If unsure, there are some formal tests that can be done to determine if someone has dementia. For example, a doctor or healthcare provider can study medical and family history, do a physical examination, and perform laboratory tests. They can evaluate changes in behavior, thinking, and abilities. Using a variety of information, a dementia diagnosis can be made with relative certainty. Of course, it can be difficult to determine the exact type of dementia, as symptoms can be quite similar, as discussed earlier.

Risk Factors of Dementia

Hopefully, there will be a cure for dementia in the future. For now, the most important thing we can do is take steps, through preventive measures, to reduce the risk of developing dementia. Prevention may also strengthen our bodies to the degree that we can further delay progression if we are ever diagnosed. We may even be able to reverse the effects to some extent.

Prevention starts with understanding the risk factors of dementia. A risk factor is a condition that increases the likelihood of developing a disease or disorder. Although a complete understanding of dementia has been elusive for the medical community, there is agreement on certain risk factors when it comes to more common types of dementia, such as Alzheimer's disease and vascular dementia.

Some of the risk factors can be controlled by actions we take, so they no longer increase our risk. Others cannot be controlled and are just part of life. Even if we cannot control all of the risk factors of dementia, we may still be able to remove the trigger, or triggers, that ultimately lead to the condition.

The following risk factors of dementia can be controlled, or modified, through changes in behavior, or medical treatments [11, 12, 13].

Risk Factors that CAN be Controlled or Modified:

• **Smoking cigarettes** – People who smoke increase their risk of developing Alzheimer's disease by almost fifty percent. The risk increases for other types of dementia as well, including vascular dementia.

• **High blood pressure** – People with chronic high blood pressure (hypertension) are more likely to develop dementia. In particular, vascular dementia risk increases, largely due to the effect of high blood pressure on the heart and arteries, and due to the increased risk of stroke. Hypertension can also be caused by other risk factors of dementia. These include an unhealthy diet, excessive alcohol consumption, lack of physical activity, sleeping disorders (e.g. sleep apnea), unhealthy weight gain, and misuse of certain medications.

• **Diabetes** – Type 2 diabetes is a chronic disease that increases the risk of dementia, including Alzheimer's disease and vascular dementia. Type 2 diabetes can be caused by other risk factors of dementia, including lack of physical activity, unhealthy weight gain, family history and genetics, high blood pressure, and high cholesterol [14].

• **High cholesterol** – People with high blood cholesterol (high LDL cholesterol) have a higher risk of dementia. In addition, high cholesterol contributes to a higher risk of cardiovascular disease (heart disease). High cholesterol can be caused by other risk factors of dementia, including an unhealthy diet, lack of physical activity, unhealthy weight gain, family history and genetics, and age.

● **Obesity** – Obesity is implicated in a number of chronic diseases and conditions, including diabetes and high blood pressure, both of which increase dementia risk. Obesity may also increase the risk of multiple types of dementia directly. Unhealthy weight gain is typically caused by an unhealthy diet and a lack of physical activity. Certain medications, certain health conditions (e.g. hormone problems), and family history and genetics can also contribute to obesity.

● **Lack of physical activity** – This is related to obesity and also increases the risk of diabetes and high blood pressure, among other chronic diseases and conditions. By extension, lack of physical activity increases dementia risk.

● **Excessive Alcohol** – Drinking alcohol in moderation generally lowers risk. Excessive consumption increases risk. Excessive alcohol consumption can also lead to a vitamin B1 (Thiamine) deficiency, which is associated with Wernicke-Korsakoff Syndrome [15].

● **Depression** – People with a history of depression, or those that suffer from depression later in life, may develop dementia as a result. As it turns out, depression is also a common early symptom of dementia.

● **Head injury** – Severe head injuries, or repeated head injuries, increase the risk of dementia, including Alzheimer's, even if many years have passed since the original injury. There is also an increased risk of diminishing brain function in the near-term [16].

● **Low level of education** – More education decreases the risk of dementia later in life. By extension, lifelong learning activities also help to reduce risk. A larger, and more active, brain is more resilient to dementia-related damage. This increased resilience is called **cognitive reserve** [17].

● **Misuse or overuse of certain medications** – Some over the counter and prescription medications can increase risk of dementia [18]. For example, long-term use of anticholinergic drugs, such as Benadryl, Demerol,

Dimetapp, Dramamine, Paxil, Unisom, and VESIcare, appears to have a negative effect on memory, verbal reasoning, planning, and problem solving.

• **Excessive stress** – Stress is largely ignored as a risk factor. However, a persistent high level of stress can increase the risk of a number of chronic diseases and conditions, including dementia.

• **Lack of sleep** – Insufficient sleep or poor sleep quality can increase the risk of multiple chronic diseases and conditions, including dementia. It can also contribute to other associated risk factors, such as obesity and stress.

*　　*　　*

There are a variety of **potential risk factors** that are more difficult to define and more difficult to prove when it comes to direct causation. Still, these risk factors as listed below should be avoided if possible, especially if the cost to address them is low. Future research should provide more evidence, eventually.

• **Exposure to pollutants in the air** – Chemical pollutants in the air can build up in our bodies, and in our brains, over time. Research suggests a possible link to a variety of diseases and conditions, including dementia [19].

• **Exposure to toxic chemicals** – There are chemicals all around us. For example, household chemicals, which are perceived as harmless, are often used improperly. This can increase exposure to unsafe levels, and possibly result in increased risk [20].

• **Exposure to cellphone radiation** – Prolonged exposure to radiation from cellphones, in the vicinity of the head, may affect the brain in subtle ways over the long term. When neurons communicate with each other, they do so through electrical and chemical impulses. The radiation emitted from cellphones is an electromagnetic field, albeit a relatively weak one. There is evidence that stronger fields can increase risk of dementia [21]. However, electromagnetic fields of any strength have the potential to stimulate or otherwise affect brain cells in some way over time. We do not fully understand what the long term effects are.

● **Overuse of technological aids** – This is related to an earlier risk factor involving low levels of education. Technology has drastically changed our behavior. Reliance on technological aids, particularly computers and smartphones, can result in less mental stimulation over a long period of time. If you stop using your brain for doing everyday calculations or information processing, you may end up with a smaller, less active, brain, and one that is less resilient to dementia.

*   *   *

There are a few risk factors, listed below, that cannot be controlled or modified through behavioral changes or medical treatments [11]. However, we may still be able to reduce the severity of these risk factors indirectly by minimizing the effects of the other risk factors highlighted above.

Risk Factors that CANNOT be Controlled or Modified:

● **Age** – Age increases the risk of a range of chronic diseases and conditions, dementia among them. There is no way to reverse this process.

● **Family history and genetics** – Our genetic makeup influences how susceptible we are to certain chronic diseases and conditions, including dementia. People with a family history of dementia should probably increase the number of medical screenings, starting in mid-life, and take additional steps to decrease risk.

*   *   *

Even though we can't change our age or our genes, our environment and our behavior can cause specific changes in our bodies that can either trigger or stave off dementia many years in the future. For example, in reference to Alzheimer's, genetics certainly plays a factor, but it is believed that a combination of risk factors contributes collectively to an increased risk. There are many variables at play. Therefore, it is important to do everything we can, without delay, to minimize the risk factors that we can control. This is our chance to influence the outcome.

Fighting Back against Dementia

There are certain measures we can take at home, with our families, to help prevent dementia. In reference to prevention, we have already covered the many risk factors of dementia. If we simply focus on avoiding these risk factors, we can reduce our risk dramatically.

However, there is more that we can do. We can stimulate the brain to make it more resilient. We may even be able to regain some of our mental abilities, despite suffering seemingly irreversible damage. So, even if someone has dementia already, certain activities can help mitigate or reverse the effects, particularly in the earlier stages.

The remainder of this book will cover these measures and more. To fight back against dementia, consider the following brain health imperatives.

● **Follow a healthy diet** – Our diet plays a role in chronic disease prevention, and reduces risk across the board. It is also important for maintaining brain health. Therefore, we should start by following a healthy diet. This does not have to be a complicated endeavor. For more information, refer to the chapter on Healthy Eating.

● **Consider dietary supplements, but only use them as a last resort** – Although not recommended as a primary source of nutrients, some supplements may possibly be effective for preventing and mitigating symptoms of dementia in limited circumstances. Even so, nothing replaces a healthy diet. The exception is when supplements are used to treat known vitamin deficiencies. More information can be found in the chapter on Dietary Supplements.

• **Improve digestive health to improve brain health** – The link between the digestive system and the brain is not fully understood. Based on what we know however, digestive health influences how we think and feel and is of paramount importance when discussing brain health. For more information, refer to the chapter on Digestive Health.

• **Increase the amount of exercise and physical activity** – Exercise decreases the risk of dementia. It improves blood circulation in the body and brain, and is also a form of brain stimulation. For more information, refer to the chapters on Aerobic Exercise and Physical Activities.

• **Reinforce the brain through a variety of mental and physical activities** – Brain stimulation activities may increase our mental capacities and can be used to help rehabilitate those who are suffering from dementia symptoms. More information can be found in the chapters on Do-It-Yourself Brain Stimulation, Physical Activities, Social Activities, New Experiences, Memory Training, Sensory Stimulation, and Brain Training.

• **Get plenty of sleep** – An adequate amount of quality sleep is extremely important for general health. It also helps the brain rest and repair, and as a result, decreases the risk of developing dementia. For more information, see the chapter on Adequate Sleep.

• **Minimize exposure to environmental chemicals** – Chemicals are everywhere in our environment. Some of them are known to be toxic and others have the potential to be toxic. And for some, the long-term effects are unknown. Low-cost avoidance measures should be used to minimize exposure to these chemicals until further research can be done to confirm their safety. For more information, see the chapter on Environmental Chemical Avoidance.

• **Avoid other risk factors through behavior** – There are a few risk factors that can be largely avoided with a change in behavior. Others can be avoided by seeking help when needed. In both cases, it is up to us to take action for the sake of long-term brain health. More information can be found in the chapter on Lifestyle Changes.

Healthy Eating

A healthy diet is extremely important when it comes to general health and increased lifespan. In fact, a number of known health problems can be largely prevented by a healthy diet alone. Many of these health problems also happen to be risk factors for dementia, including high blood pressure, diabetes, and obesity.

In addition to the many health benefits, a healthy diet ensures that you are getting the nutrients you need for healthy brain function. Furthermore, some nutritional deficiencies can raise your risk of developing dementia, especially later in life. There is simply no better way to prevent these deficiencies than to eat more of the right foods and less of the wrong ones.

There are many diets that are designed to serve a particular purpose, such as weight loss. Others promise to solve certain problems related to health, such as high blood pressure or high cholesterol. There is even a diet called the MIND diet (Mediterranean-DASH Intervention for Neurodegenerative Delay diet) for preventing Alzheimer's disease, in particular [22]. It combines aspects of two popular heart-healthy diets, the Mediterranean diet and the DASH diet.

However, when it comes down to the basics, most of these diets, including the MIND diet, follow the same basic patterns and recommendations. In general, to obtain all the nutrients you need to prevent chronic diseases, including brain diseases related to dementia, you need to eat a variety of nutrient-dense foods in all food groups. To achieve these aims, incorporate the following into your diet [23].

● **Fruits and vegetables** – This group includes fruits, especially whole fruits, and a variety of vegetables including dark green, red and orange vegetables, and beans and peas.

● **Whole grains** – This group includes whole grain breads (e.g. whole grain sliced bread, bagels, muffins, rolls, pitas, and tortillas), whole grain cereals (e.g. oats, barley, buckwheat, and shredded wheat), brown rice, and whole wheat pastas. Use whole grains to replace refined grains, such as white flour, white rice, and white bread, whenever possible.

• **Non-fat or low-fat dairy products** – This group includes milk, yogurt, cheese, sour cream, and fortified soy drinks.

• **Healthy protein foods** – This group includes a variety of healthy protein sources, such as seafood, lean meats, poultry, eggs, beans, peas, nuts, seeds, and soy products.

• **Healthy Oils** – This group includes olive, canola, coconut, soy, corn, sesame, peanut, flaxseed, and other vegetable oils.

*   *   *

These foods contain vitamins, minerals, and other nutrients that are important to maintain overall health, including brain health.

To further increase the health benefits of food as it relates to prevention of dementia, consider the following additional nutritional guidelines.

• **Limit saturated fats and *trans* fats, added sugars, and sodium** – Consuming these nutrients in excess amounts can lead to chronic diseases and conditions that are linked to dementia, including diabetes, obesity, and high blood pressure. You should be able to find information on these nutrients, including the percent daily value, on the food nutrition label of most products.

• **Increase the consumption of certain brain-boosting foods** – As specified in the MIND diet, brain-boosting foods may provide additional brain health benefits. So, consume more fish, poultry, olive oil, wine (in moderation), nuts, berries, beans, and whole grains, in addition to vegetables of all colors [24]. All of these foods are included in the prior food recommendations, except for wine.

• **Limit the consumption of heavily-processed foods** – Heavily processed foods, such as processed meats, snack foods, and some convenience foods, such as microwave dinners and fast food meals, typically contain a lot of artificial ingredients and are largely devoid of nutrients.

• **Eat as many different types of food as possible** – This will ensure that you are getting a variety of nutrients in your diet. Eat different types of foods, try different brands, buy fresh and frozen foods, and eat cooked and raw foods. Different types of food will have different nutrient compositions and consuming a variety will help avoid nutrient deficiencies that may result from eating only one type of food.

Dietary Supplements

The easiest way to consume the nutrients you need for healthy brain function is by following a healthy diet. However, many people use other methods to get the nutrients that they need. This is usually in the form of nutritional supplements.

Nutritional supplements provide an alternative method for dealing with nutritional deficiencies. There is no benefit to consuming more of a certain nutrient than your body needs or produces on its own. Some supplement manufacturers and distributors promise certain health benefits, but these benefits are largely unproven.

The bottom line is that supplements should only be taken as a last resort. If you are healthy, you probably don't need them. And, unless you are prescribed a supplement for a known nutritional deficiency, you should probably avoid them entirely. Instead, focus on eating healthy foods.

There are a variety of supplements that may help address nutrient deficiencies that are related to dementia. Some may or may not improve brain function. If you still feel you must take supplements due to an inadequate diet or some other reason, the following list is a good place to start [25, 26]. All of these supplements are available over-the-counter or online.

Nutritional supplements:

● **B vitamins** – B vitamins, such as Biotin, B1, B2, B6, B12, and folic acid are important for brain function, so supplementation may reduce the risk of dementia. B vitamins may also help relieve symptoms of dementia, including Alzheimer's disease. For Wernicke-Korsakoff syndrome in particular, supplementing with vitamin B1 (thiamine), both decreases risk and relieves symptoms.

● **Vitamin D** – Supplementing with vitamin D may reduce the risk of dementia, including Alzheimer's disease [27].

● **Coenzyme Q10** – This antioxidant supplement may help increase oxygen levels in the brain. Consequently, it may prevent, or at least slow the progression of dementia.

● **Zinc** – Zinc deficiency is common in elderly. Supplementing with zinc may improve memory and increase resiliency to dementia.

● **Phosphatidylserine** – This supplement may help improve memory and relieve mild symptoms of dementia.

● **Vitamin E** – This vitamin, combined with certain prescribed drugs, may slow Alzheimer's disease progression.

● **L-arginine** – This amino acid supplement may help increase blood flow to the brain. Increased blood flow may help relieve symptoms of dementia, particularly vascular dementia.

● **Omega 3 fatty acids** – Supplementing with Omega 3 fatty acids may reduce risk overall.

• **Melatonin** – When combined with regular physical exercise, melatonin may relieve some symptoms of dementia, including anxiety, depression, and behavioral problems. It may also increase resiliency to dementia.

• **Creatine** – This amino acid helps provide energy for muscles. Consequently, supplementing with creatine may help slow Parkinson's disease progression.

Herbal supplements:

• **Ginkgo (*Ginkgo biloba*)** – This plant extract may help relieve symptoms of dementia, including Alzheimer's disease and vascular dementia.

• **Huperzine A (*Huperzia serrata*)** – This plant chemical may improve memory for those suffering from Alzheimer's disease and vascular dementia.

• **Lemon balm (*Melissa officinalis*)** – This herb may help improve brain function for those with Alzheimer's disease.

• **Brahmi (*Bacopa monnieri*)** – This herb may help improve brain function and learning ability. Consequently, it may increase resiliency to dementia.

• **American ginseng (*Panax quinquefolium*)** – This herb may help increase blood flow to the brain, which may, in turn, help relieve symptoms of dementia, including vascular dementia.

• **Vinpocetine (*Vinca minor*)** – This herb may also help increase blood flow to the brain.

*   *   *

Note that supplements can interfere with prescription medication and may also have serious side effects depending on the dosage used. So, be sure to follow the recommendations on the label at the very least. It may also be wise to consult your doctor or healthcare provider before taking them.

Digestive Health

Your digestive system, also known as your gut, contains numerous tiny microorganisms, including bacteria and fungi. We cannot see them, but they are there in the gastrointestinal tract, numbering in the trillions. Unlike some other microorganisms, they don't cause illness. Their presence is actually beneficial and necessary, not only for digestive health, but for overall health as well. For example, these microorganisms help digest food, create essential nutrients, secrete important chemicals, and support our immune system to fight infection. We simply cannot live without them.

At the same time, research is uncovering important links between the brain and these microorganisms. For example, they may influence, strongly, how we think and feel [28]. Research is also uncovering their critical role in disorders such as anxiety and depression. It just so happens that such disorders are risk factors for dementia.

The microorganisms in your gut communicate with the brain through chemical signals, as well as through the nervous system [29]. Some of these chemicals (e.g. dopamine) are implicated in the development of dementia. Research is ongoing to confirm these links, but it is not a stretch to say that the state of your digestive health is influential when it comes to brain health and the development of dementia.

To improve overall health and possibly prevent dementia, take the following steps to improve digestive health.

• **Follow a healthy diet** – Eat a variety of nutrient-dense foods in all food groups, as previously discussed. An unhealthy diet consisting of heavily-processed foods may increase inflammation in the gut and weaken the immune system. And, it certainly will affect the composition of microorganisms there. By eating a healthy, varied diet, you increase the diversity of good bacteria and allow them to flourish. This supports digestive health, and by extension, supports brain health.

- **Eat food sources of prebiotics** [30] – Prebiotics are nutrients that feed beneficial bacteria. By eating foods containing these nutrients, you create a better environment for bacteria to live and multiply. Examples of ideal foods containing prebiotics include bananas, berries, legumes, garlic, onions, leeks, whole grains, nuts, and seeds. Examples of ideal food ingredients, as shown on nutrition labels, include acacia gum, inulin, lactulose, arabinose, fructooligosaccharides, galactooligosaccharides, maltodextrin, and wheat dextrin.

- **Eat food sources of probiotics** [31] – Probiotics are live bacteria, the same type of good bacteria that are typically found in the gut. By eating foods containing probiotics, you may be able to replenish some of the good bacteria. Examples of common food sources of probiotics include cultured yogurt, kefir, sauerkraut, kimchi, miso, and cultured (non-pasteurized) milk.

*   *   *

There are, of course, prebiotic and probiotic supplements on the market. Although not ideal when compared to food, these supplements may be beneficial for improving digestive health. They are often used to quickly replenish gut bacteria when taking medication or antibiotics, both of which can kill off good bacteria, potentially causing digestive problems.

Aerobic Exercise

Regular physical exercise is one of the most powerful tools you have in the fight against dementia. Studies show that greater fitness levels, particularly aerobic fitness, relates to stronger brain function in older adults [32]. Exercise can lead to greater resiliency, preventing mental decline. It can improve circulation by promoting the creation of new blood vessels and can increase the overall size of the brain, especially in areas responsible for memory and thinking [33]. In addition, regular exercise counteracts multiple risk factors for dementia, including obesity and diabetes.

Regular exercise has a number of other health benefits as well. Exercise is proven to improve mental health and mood. Exercise even improves sleep and helps to cope with stress, which is yet another risk factor for dementia. With all of these benefits, and there are others, physical activity in the form of regular exercise should be one of the top priorities for someone looking to prevent and reverse the effects of dementia.

In order for aerobic exercise to be effective, it must have a sufficient level of intensity. Ideal aerobic exercise falls into two basic categories, moderate and high-intensity. Examples of moderate-intensity aerobic exercise include cross-country hiking, swimming, jogging, low impact aerobics, dancing, walking, and yoga. Examples of high-intensity aerobic exercise include running, bicycling, high-impact aerobics, swimming laps, and sports such as tennis.

For exercise to be classified as regular exercise, an activity must take at least 10 minutes at a time. And depending on the intensity of exercise, you could increase or decrease the amount of time you spend exercising and get the same health benefits.

According to the Physical Activity Guidelines for Americans [34], the recommended amount of exercise, based on intensity, is as follows.

Moderate-intensity exercise:

● **Recommended** – Accumulate a minimum of **150 minutes of moderate-intensity exercise or 2.5 hours per week,** according to your schedule. For example, you could do 50 minutes of walking per day, 3 times per week, or spread it out even further by doing 30 minutes of walking, 5 times per week. The total amount of exercise should add up to 150 minutes.

● **For increased health benefits** – Accumulate **300 minutes of moderate-intensity exercise or 5 hours per week** according to your schedule. For example, you could do 60 minutes of walking per day, 5 times per week or you could try splitting it up during the day by doing 30 minutes of walking in the morning and 30 minutes of walking at night.

High-intensity exercise:

● **Recommended** – Accumulate a minimum of **75 minutes of high-intensity exercise or 1.25 hours per week**. For example, you could do 25 minutes per day of running, 3 times per week, or spread it out even further by doing 15 minutes of running per day, 5 times per week.

● **For increased health benefits** – Accumulate **150 minutes of high-intensity exercise or 2.5 hours per week**. For example, you could do 30 minutes of bicycling per day, 5 times per week or split up activities during different parts of the day.

*   *   *

Customize your schedule according to your needs, but make sure you get the recommended amount of exercise per week.

The key to keeping up a regular exercise program is to do activities you enjoy. Exercising consistently over a longer period of time will maximize health benefits. If you are suffering from chronic pain that makes exercise difficult, a healthcare provider or specialist may be able to find exercises that you can perform.

Later, we will cover how other physical activities, not normally associated with exercise, can improve brain health.

Do-It-Yourself Brain Stimulation

Brain cells communicate with each other and form new connections based on the activities we engage in, our interaction with the environment, and how we behave over time. Consequently, the brain reorganizes and continues to develop over the course of one's life. Thus, if we intentionally stimulate the brain in certain ways, we may also be able to create new connections, or new channels of communication, between brain cells. This is based on a concept called neuroplasticity [35]. Such brain reorganization can happen throughout various regions of the brain, at any age.

Even as brain cells die due to injury or disease, we can reestablish connections to some extent, and we should make every effort to do so, no matter what condition we are in. As stated previously, the brain is a massively connected network of brain cells. The interconnectivity of the brain is vast and brain cells are connected to each other across regions as well as within regions. Research has confirmed that even if brain cells die in one region of the brain, **brain cells in another region can compensate for lost functionality in that region**. This can even occur when entire regions of the brain have been severely damaged by stroke.

Leveraging the concept of neuroplasticity and the interconnectivity of the brain, we can stimulate the brain in a variety of ways in order to make it more resilient to dementia. To accomplish this and more, consider the following strategies.

● **Create new connections through challenging activities and new experiences** – Challenging activities and new experiences are highly effective when it comes to brain reorganization and may result in more connections across different regions of the brain. By stimulating the brain in this way, we can increase our mental capabilities. We actively learn new ways to solve problems and perform complex tasks. And of course, increasing the number of connections increases cognitive reserve, which helps increase resiliency to dementia-induced damage.

• **Keep active to protect the brain from loss** – We also need to continue to engage in activities that we do regularly and expect to do more of in the future. By overlooking and discontinuing such menial activities, the associated connections become inactive and grow weaker. So, for example, we need to continue to do basic household chores such as setting the table, folding the clothes, raking the lawn, and making the bed. The best way to preserve function is to keep on doing it. More practice will make those connections stronger.

• **Stimulate as many different areas of the brain as possible** – There is no panacea for dementia, and every individual is different. In other words, there is no software product, exercise program, or specialized activity that is going to magically work to prevent or cure it. Therefore, it is best not to overspecialize, especially if an activity only focuses on one area of the brain. Since the brain is interconnected within and across regions, we need to expand our selection of activities to recruit brain cells from all regions. Better yet, we should try to find activities that stimulate these regions simultaneously and then do a variety of such activities with plenty of overlap. Such an approach is more effective than focusing on only one area of the brain.

• **Engage in activities that are enjoyable over the long-term** – If you cannot keep up an activity over the long term, you may eventually lose the associated functionality that the activity provides. If you don't use it, you will lose it, especially if you are at risk for dementia. A fancy training program is not going to work if you can't, or don't want to, keep it up. Make your life more personalized. Do a variety of stimulating activities that you enjoy the most, and keep on doing them.

*   *   *

The next few chapters will give you some ideas on how to stimulate the brain based on the above strategies. Many of these activities will overlap in with respect to the type of brain stimulation. This is ideal and necessary in order to increase resiliency. Keep in mind that these suggestions just represent the tip of the iceberg on what is possible.

Physical Activities

For brain health, as well as general health, it is advisable to do as much physical activity as possible. Even if aerobic exercise is not possible or if you live a largely sedentary lifestyle, some form of physical activity can be done throughout the day, by mixing it in with other activities. In fact, certain activities that you engage in regularly, such as household chores and yardwork, may be considered strenuous exercise. For example, carrying boxes, washing the car, shoveling snow, digging or spading dirt, gardening, raking leaves, and painting the house can all be considered aerobic exercise depending on intensity.

Aside from the obvious health benefits, physical activities also stimulate multiple regions of the brain simultaneously. For example, many of the activities mentioned previously require thinking and planning (frontal lobe), muscle control (frontal lobe), spatial perception and sense of touch (parietal lobe), sequencing of actions (temporal lobe), and visual processing (occipital lobe). Such physical activities not only help to prevent dementia, but they can also be therapeutic for those who are exhibiting early signs.

Consider the following suggestions on how to include stimulating physical activities throughout the day, at home or at work. This is not a complete list.

• **Do more household chores** – Activities such as doing the grocery shopping, organizing the canned goods, washing the dishes, setting the table, folding the clothes, and cleaning the house may seem like a burden. However, these activities are likely to be even more beneficial than other brain stimulation methods. As a form of practice, they help maintain quality of life and help preserve independence. Participate in as many of these activities as you can, and do more of it as you get older. Naturally, if someone is already suffering from dementia, some of these activities may not be appropriate or may need to be scaled back for safety reasons.

• **Do more walking** – Squeeze in short walks whenever and wherever you can. For example, the next time you go shopping, park your vehicle farther away from the entrance. Or, purposely take a longer route on foot than you normally would when you go somewhere (e.g. a store in a mall or a friend's house down the street).

• **Take the stairs** – If you are able, try to take the stairs rather than the elevator, even if you can only manage a few floors at a time.

• **Take active mini-breaks** – While you are at work, take short physical activity breaks to walk around, stand up, or stretch. In reference to general health, these simple actions are important, especially for those who sit at a computer desk all day.

• **Spend active time with family and friends** – Instead of just sitting around to talk, catch up on events with family and friends while taking a walk together or while working together on an active hobby project. Or, spend time to play with children (e.g. throw a ball around).

• **Spend active time with pets** – Find time to walk the dog regularly, even if it is for a short while.

• **Participate in active hobbies** – Consider adopting new hobbies that involve more physical activity or allow you to work with your hands. Examples include gardening, knitting, home improvement activities, and fixing old cars.

• **Play physical video games** – If you like to play video games, mix things up by playing games on platforms that capture body motion and hand gestures as input, rather than a handheld controller.

• **Dance** – Dancing is a great form of exercise and is one of the most stimulating activities for the brain that you can do. Some studies have shown that dancing decreases risk of dementia significantly, when compared to other physical activities [36]. Dancing is even used to treat people with Parkinson's disease. Whether you go out dancing regularly, or you decide to take a few dance classes here and there, find the time to dance and do it often.

*   *   *

To maintain maximum mobility, you need to increase the amount of physical activity throughout the day, in addition to regular aerobic exercise. Remember, if the activity is simple, convenient, and fun, you are more likely to continue it over the long term. Frequent physical activity improves general health, and improves your brain health at the same time.

Social Activities

Social interaction is also important for brain health. Research has shown that increasing social interaction decreases the risk of dementia [37]. It also stimulates multiple areas of the brain simultaneously. For example, participating in a face-to-face conversation with someone requires speaking skills and concentration (frontal lobe), language skills (parietal and temporal lobe), hearing and memory (temporal lobe), and interpretation of visual information (occipital lobe).

There are other health benefits as well. Social interaction decreases stress and helps to prevent depression, both of which are risk factors. Plus, participating in social groups can encourage other healthy activities, such as exercise, learning, and exploration, including travel. Such activities counteract known dementia risk factors and stimulate the brain at the same time. So, it is no surprise that maintaining social connections (friendships) and engaging in social activities are an important part of a dementia treatment regimen.

Given the benefits, the integration of social activities should be a central part of any do-it-yourself brain stimulation program. Consider the following list of suggestions as a starting point.

• **Stay active in the workplace** – Depending on the type of work you do, staying active in the workplace can be a great way to maintain interaction with people. If you don't already have a job, an interesting seasonal or part-time position may be therapeutic, and may help to delay or even prevent dementia at the same time. In some cases, permanent retirement is a bad idea, not just because it eliminates a source of mental stimulation, but also because, for some people, it results in a significant loss of social interaction.

• **Increase social interaction in day-to-day life** – Connect with friends and family regularly on the phone and in person. And don't be afraid to start conversations with your neighbors. If there are too few opportunities to converse, take the initiative to host a social event like a neighborhood get-together or dinner party. This will stimulate the brain even further by affording an opportunity to plan activities and remember details. Get a friend or family member to help. If you are not able to connect with people in person or on the phone, try becoming more active on social media, which can serve to fill in the gaps.

• **Join clubs or groups** – Clubs or groups provide an opportunity to engage in discussion, play games, enjoy art, learn new hobbies, enjoy food, and make new friends. For example, joining a book club presents an opportunity to read, exchange book ideas, and discuss them with others in the group. There are plenty of options. Check social media sites to see if there are any interesting groups in your area. And if options are limited, you can join an online discussion group or forum, which can still give opportunities for interaction, as well as supplement existing in-person interactions.

• **Join a physical activity group or class** – This is a great opportunity to meet new people and stay active at the same time. Take a group exercise class in yoga, tai chi, step aerobics, or swimming. Join groups that go running or hiking on the weekends. Since dancing is highly stimulating for the brain, consider taking a ballroom dance class, which counts as a physical activity and gives you a chance to meet new people.

● **Take any adult education class** – These short classes are often available at the local university and are usually inexpensive. For example, a cooking class will stimulate the senses and provide opportunities to meet new people. A computer class may also involve social interaction, and it doubles as a brain training activity. Better yet, take a class with a friend, and you can practice what you have learned together as a memory exercise.

● **Play more social games** – Examples of socially-oriented games include trivia games, multiplayer board games, and multiplayer card games. There are online computer versions of these games as well. In addition to providing a means to connect with people, these games also serve as good brain training activities.

● **Volunteer** – Volunteering at a soup kitchen, charity event, school function, city function, or animal shelter is another great way to meet and converse with people. The chance to make a difference in the community and help others will likely improve mood, as a bonus.

New Experiences

New experiences greatly encourage brain reorganization and the formation of new connections. They can be in the form of creative hobbies, learning activities, or travel and exploration. To be more stimulating, new experiences should be novel and exciting. That way, your brain will treat them as important.

Being creative is particularly stimulating. When you do something creative, there is increased communication between different regions of the brain [38]. This is expected as you are forced to come up with new ideas and use multiple regions of the brain simultaneously to solve new problems. In the process, you have to learn new ways of doing things and correct mistakes.

This learning and repetition will make connections even stronger. Plus, increased learning, in turn, can make you even more creative, in addition to the other benefits.

It is important to stimulate the brain through new experiences to metaphorically jolt it out of its slumber from time to time. Therefore, you should get out of your comfort zone, and do something new, exciting, challenging, and creative as often as you can. The following are some suggestions for experiencing something new.

● **Find more ways to be more creative** – Put a learned skill or new hobby to work. Opportunities for creativity can come from participating in arts and crafts, house decorating, creative writing, storytelling, taking pictures or photos, playing musical instruments, painting, or any kind of problem solving. Start a new hobby or rediscover an old one. The possibilities are limitless.

● **Go back to school or learn something new** – Taking education classes is a widely-available method of stimulating your brain. Consider going back to school part-time to expand your mental capacities and learn new skills. Many universities have continuing education classes or online programs that allow you to explore new subjects, without enrolling in a degree program. Taking a class in a new subject area opens up new possibilities, new experiences, new knowledge, and new relationships.

● **Travel someplace exotic** – Travel to places you've never been before with family and friends. You will meet new people, experience new sights and sounds, and challenge your brain. If you are on a budget, explore new parts of your city or state.

● **Explore your local community** – Look for new things to do in your local community. Shop at a new store, go to a flea market, try a new restaurant, or check out local events and conferences. Bring family and friends to make the experience more fulfilling.

• **Surf the web randomly on various topics** – We spend a lot of time online, so, try to mix things up a bit when you spend time in front of the computer. Don't just go to the same sites over and over. By visiting new sites, you will expand your knowledge, have fun, and likely discover new opportunities for growth. There is one caveat for this type of activity: do not give out your personal information or buy anything online unless you trust the site you are visiting.

• **Change your routine** – Try mixing up your routine with respect to your schedule and activities. Try doing your errands on a different day. Pick a different night to socialize or see a movie. Switch up your regular routine and strive for variation when the opportunity presents itself.

• **Change your environment** – Try reorganizing your home or office. Rearrange the furniture from time to time. Such changes can be invigorating and result in new experiences. Sometimes, actually moving to a new address or a new part of town is just what you need to shake things up. If none of this is an option for you, consider virtual reality technology as a way to immerse yourself in a virtual, and challenging, world. It is not as stimulating as real life, but soon you will be able to travel almost anywhere in the comfort of your own home using only a headset. Virtual reality equipment is becoming cheaper over time and certain applications are being considered as stimulating activities for dementia patients.

Memory Training

Utilizing memory involves storing and remembering information and experiences. Research has shown that memory-related training activities can relieve symptoms of dementia and potentially make the brain more resilient in the future [39]. So, it is worth engaging in such activities, especially in a fun way, to help preserve function.

The process of using your memory stimulates multiple areas of the brain, including the frontal, parietal, and temporal lobes. By using various methods to encourage recall of past experiences and then sharing those memories with others, you are essentially participating in something called **reminiscence therapy**. This type of therapy has been used to treat dementia patients to relieve symptoms and improve mood [40]. You can perform such therapy at home, on your own.

The key to memory training of any type is practice. Formal memory training methods can be effective, but those are not likely to be as much fun and may require supervision to keep them up. When performed on your own, you need to choose activities that are enjoyable, exciting, and diverse enough to keep your interest over time. You should use memory aides that involve all five senses if possible. This will help trigger memories, old and new. Getting family and friends involved will help even more, and will further encourage recall.

The following are ideas for stimulating the brain to preserve memory. The same type of activities may also improve memory function.

• **Decorate your home or office** – Surround yourself with decorations that serve as memory aides. Hang up pictures of family, friends, and familiar scenery on the walls or display them on a shelf. If all of your photos are on your computer or smartphone, acquire digital photo frames so you can display them properly. Organize decorative items on shelves and coffee tables, including souvenirs and other display items. Show off some of your favorite indoor plants and flowers. Display your favorite colors. Put up decorations that remind you of happy memories that will encourage storytelling when people come over to visit.

• **Create a memory scrapbook** – Collect a variety of things that will trigger memories of the past, such as pictures, books, videos, audio recordings, music samples, and old food recipes. Collect such items in a scrap book, store them on a computer, or share them on social media. Then, review them periodically and relive those memories. Better yet, share them with friends and family.

36

• **Play trivia games** – Trivia games are ideal for learning and remembering new facts and other pieces of information. Such games are often social activities as well, which is a bonus.

• **Make television watching active instead of passive** – Television does not have to be a passive activity. For example, after watching a television show or movie, try to remember the details of what you saw. Create a synopsis in your head, recall the characters, or play the critic and discuss the plot points with friends and family. Alternatively, watch a thought-provoking movie or documentary, and try to remember what you have learned afterwards.

• **Learn a new language** – Studying a foreign language is a memory-intensive activity. Take a class or join a language learning group if it helps to keep up with the activity over time. Alternatively, focus on improving the vocabulary of your native language. As you hear and read new words, write them down and look them up online or in a dictionary, and review them from time to time.

• **Challenge yourself during social interactions** – At social events, try to remember the names of people you meet. Engage in conversation by telling jokes that you heard, share memories from the past, discuss current events, and exchange knowledge. If person-to-person interaction is not possible, social media is a great way to engage in the same kinds of activities.

• **Keep an idea notebook or journal** – Keep a notebook or recording device with you at all times. Record your important thoughts, experiences, interactions, or creative ideas whenever they come up. Include pictures or sketches when you can. Consider using a voice or video recorder. Store them and then periodically review them to relive memories and revisit ideas.

Sensory Stimulation

Sensory stimulation involves the use of one or more of the senses including sight, smell, hearing, taste, and touch. Activities involving sight stimulate the occipital lobe, hearing and smell stimulates the temporal lobe, and touch and taste stimulates the parietal lobe. Ideal activities should stimulate multiple areas of the brain simultaneously. Utilizing all five senses may also serve as a form of memory training, by helping to recall past memories based on experiences involving those senses.

The following are examples of sensory stimulation activities. Try to come up with some of your own, and make sure to use as many senses as possible.

● **Take a walk outside in nature** – This is a great physical activity and can boost mood as well. It stimulates multiple senses. Remember to focus your attention on the various sights, sounds, and smells that you encounter. If you do not have a park nearby, try exploring your own neighborhood by taking a different route or exploring a different area. If you are uncomfortable doing so, take a friend or family member with you and make it a social activity.

● **Take up gardening** – Gardening has been mentioned as an activity before, but it is worth mentioning again for the purpose of sensory stimulation. When you are gardening, you are working with your hands and, in the process, feeling the soil and materials. You can plant new crops, herbs, and flowers and experience the new smells and textures as you do so. You can also enjoy the sights, sounds, and fresh air of the outdoors. Gardening is a physical activity as well, so it serves as a great all-around brain stimulation experience.

● **Enjoy the taste and smell of new food** – Go to a new restaurant and try a new type of food. Explore the menu at your favorite restaurant and try a new dish. Even better, be adventurous and use a new recipe in the kitchen. This type of activity is perfect for stimulating the brain using taste, smell, and sight.

- **Enjoy different types of music** – Listen to all types of music. Sing along if you can. Or, learn to read and play different types of music using a musical instrument. If you've never played a musical instrument before, taking a guitar or piano class doubles as a social activity.

- **Enjoy hobby activities that involve working with your hands** – Almost anything involving arts and crafts works as a sensory stimulation activity. Examples include painting, drawing or sketching, pottery, sculpting, model building, and knitting.

- **Get a therapeutic massage** – Massages have many other health benefits in addition to stimulating sense of touch. Essential oils and aromatherapy are often used as part of the experience, so you are also stimulating your sense of smell. As an alternative, try using water (hydrotherapy) as a form of massage and sensory stimulation. Swimming pools and whirlpools provide light pressure from circulating water. Water jets from hot tubs, Jacuzzis, and showers provide even more pressure. As a bonus, the temperature of the water and steam from pools, tubs, and saunas provide additional stimulation.

Brain Training

Brain training programs are marketed to increase intelligence, problem-solving skills, concentration, and memory. They often involve specialized computer applications, flashcards, puzzles, or games. Whether or not they can increase intelligence and improve other mental capabilities as advertised is a subject of debate [41]. However, there is evidence that suggests such activities can help mitigate symptoms of dementia and increase resilience [39]. If you enjoy using these specialized programs, they are worth looking into. For the rest of us, brain training activities may need to be more engaging, less boring, and easier to do over the long term. So, it is important to find activities that you enjoy personally.

Do-it-yourself brain training can be done almost anywhere, including at home, at work, or even during a commute. Taken together, such activities stimulate all areas of the brain. For example, they involve solving problems (frontal lobe), making connections (parietal lobe), processing language (temporal, parietal lobes), organizing information (temporal lobe), perceiving spatial relationships (parietal lobe), and interpreting colors (occipital lobe). You don't need complicated software or special training programs to do brain training exercises, although there are companies that specialize in developing such programs, as mentioned before. Just imagine things you enjoy doing that are challenging in some way.

The following are ideas for brain training activities to get you started. This is not a complete list, so try to come up with some of your own activities, and don't be afraid to mix them up for variety.

• **Play number games or puzzles** – Examples include Japanese puzzles such as Sudoku, and Magic Squares. Such games or puzzles can be found in the newspaper, at a bookstore, or online for free. Bingo is another number game that doubles as an enjoyable social activity.

• **Do more arithmetic in your head or on paper** – We rely too much on technological aids, such as smartphones and calculators, to do all of our calculations for us. Try solving problems by doing basic arithmetic (e.g. addition and subtraction) in your head first and then use a device to check your answer.

• **Play word games and puzzles** – Examples include crossword puzzles and scrabble. Crossword puzzles, and other games like it, can also be found in the newspaper, at a bookstore, or online for free. Scrabble is a great problem-solving game that can be played online, but it can also be played with friends, which makes it a great social activity.

• **Do more reading** – Spend more time reading books, magazines, and newspapers. Try to switch topics from time to time. If you read fiction, take a break to read non-fiction books or magazines.

• **Play casual computer games** – Try any one of the large number of puzzle games available on the Internet. There are plenty of casual games that you can download on your smartphone or computer for free.

• **Play action video games** – Video games are getting more and more sophisticated and realistic and can be an effective brain-training tool. Action games can help improve eye-hand coordination, as well as help improve spatial and visual perception. Strategy-oriented games can help develop reasoning and problem solving skills. Role playing and related multiplayer games can help improve language and conversational skills.

• **Try mechanical puzzles** – Look for two and three-dimensional puzzles that involve working with shapes while using your hands. Examples include jigsaw puzzles, cube puzzles, and wooden puzzles.

Adequate Sleep

Now that we have explored ways to stimulate the brain, we need to give the brain a chance to rest and repair. Sleep is important for a number of reasons. First, research suggests that the brain flushes out toxins during sleep [42]. Without adequate sleep, toxins can build up in the brain, leading to damage and an increased risk of Alzheimer's disease, among other types of dementia. Second, sleep is important for long-term health. Insufficient sleep leads to risk factors that are related to dementia, including high blood pressure, diabetes, obesity, and depression [43]. Sleep even plays a role in managing stress. So if you are not getting enough sleep, you are likely experiencing increased stress, which is yet another risk factor related to dementia.

Therefore, it is safe to say that insufficient sleep can increase the risk of dementia, in addition to other chronic diseases and conditions. That is why it is extremely important to get enough sleep. The general consensus is that adults should get **seven or more hours of sleep per night** to avoid such health problems [44].

Aside from getting the recommended number of hours, the quality of sleep is also important. If you are not getting good quality sleep, you could be exposing yourself to increased risk, even as you spend more time in bed. Luckily, there are a number of things you can do to get more sleep, as well as increase the quality of that sleep.

The following guidelines, often overlooked, should help improve sleep quality unless an underlying medical condition is involved [45].

• **Follow a consistent sleep schedule** – If possible, go to bed and wake up at approximately the same time each day. An erratic sleep schedule can disrupt your circadian rhythm, which is when the body expects to sleep and when it expects to wake up.

• **Control the sound, light, and temperature in the bedroom** – Eliminate unnatural conditions that have the potential to decrease sleep quality. For example, sleep in a quiet room where there will be no noise or sound disruptions during the night. Sleep in a dark room. Use shades, blinds, or curtains if the room is too bright from outside light sources. Regulate temperature so that it stays stable throughout the night, not too cold and not too hot.

• **Double-check your medication** – If you suspect that your medication is interfering with sleep, it might be possible to modify the dosage, time of day, or even the type of medication you are using. Just be sure to check with your doctor or healthcare provider first.

• **Stop using electronic devices close to bedtime** – If you read with electronic devices before bedtime, consider substituting these e-readers, tablets, or smartphones with traditional books, when the situation allows for it. Otherwise, turn the brightness setting down as low as possible.

• **Avoid taking naps during the day** – If you must nap, try not to take one late in the day, as it may interfere with normal sleep. Also, try to limit the duration to no more than thirty minutes.

• **Watch what you eat and drink late in the day** – Avoid alcohol, caffeine, and also heavy, spicy, and sugary foods within several hours before bedtime. Caffeinated food and beverages include coffee, tea, soda, and chocolate.

• **Acquire better sleeping apparatus** – If you suffer from pain that interferes with sleep, consider acquiring a better mattress, or a sleep apparatus, that provides better support and body alignment.

*   *   *

If you cannot correct a sleep problem quickly, you should consult your doctor or healthcare provider as soon as possible to diagnose and fix the problem. Conditions such as insomnia and sleep apnea are treatable conditions that are quite common in the elderly population. The longer you wait, the more you risk compounding a lack of sleep with other health problems that may surface as a result, increasing your risk of dementia in the process.

Environmental Chemical Avoidance

Chemicals exist all around us. Some of them are man-made and others exist naturally in our environment. Some chemicals, intentionally or not, are distributed in the air, water, and food. Many are embedded in building materials and are mixed into household products of all types. Most of these chemicals appear to be harmless, but some of them are known to be toxic and have the potential to negatively impact health.

It is difficult to prove the long-term health effects of such chemicals. However, even in trace amounts, they can build up in our bodies, and in our brains, over time. Even then, these chemicals may give no indication of damage in the short-term. The danger to our health is not obvious.

There are legitimate concerns about such chemicals and whether or not they increase the risk of certain brain disorders, dementia among them. For example, some studies have suggested that air pollution, from automobile emissions and industrial processes, contributes to a decline in thinking and memory skills, as well as increased risk of dementia [19]. Other studies show that long-term exposure to pesticides can lead to a similar decline [46]. The direct link between such chemicals and dementia in many cases is not definitive, but the case is getting stronger as more research is conducted [21]. Regardless, it is entirely possible that subtle effects on the brain can combine with other risk factors, such as age and family history, to trigger the development of dementia later in life.

Many researchers are also becoming more concerned about other seemingly harmless chemicals, such as those found in food, plastics, furniture, cookware, cans, carpets, electronics, and cleaning products, and even some personal care products. These chemicals are literally everywhere. And some of these everyday chemicals have the potential to affect brain development in children [20].

As we age, it becomes more difficult for our bodies to remove these chemicals and they tend to linger. And in adults, especially older adults, it is not unreasonable to assume that they can increase the risk of developing dementia. Even worse, because they build up over time, reversing the effects of dementia can be that much harder.

If we can minimize exposure to such chemicals at low cost, we should make every effort to do so. We can try to avoid using such products, but in most cases, this is not practical. We simply do not know for sure which chemicals we are exposed to and which of those chemicals are toxic. Instead, we should use some common sense to limit exposure to all environmental chemicals.

We can start with obvious measures, such as drinking filtered water and keeping surfaces free of dust. However, there are a few commonly overlooked areas that we should pay attention to if we want to decrease potential exposure. The following suggestions do not make up a complete list, but they can help reduce risk significantly when it comes to brain health.

• **Improve air quality inside the home** – We can't do much about air pollution outside the home, but we can improve the air quality inside the home. Poor air circulation and combustible byproducts are the main problems. To minimize indoor air pollution, especially from the largest sources, make sure that ventilation and air exchange systems are filtered and working properly. Periodically check to make sure that chimneys, ducts, and pipes are clean, sealed, and properly functioning. Make sure that gas ranges and heaters are venting outdoors without obstruction. Finally, try to limit secondhand smoke from cigarettes by restricting smoking activities to outdoor areas.

• **Minimize pesticide usage and exposure** – Some fruits and vegetables typically have a higher concentration of pesticide residue than others. Consider going organic for some fruits and vegetables, including strawberries, apples, nectarines, peaches, celery, grapes, cherries, spinach, tomatoes, sweet bell peppers, cherry tomatoes, cucumbers, leafy greens, and hot peppers [47]. When growing your own food, use nonchemical pest control methods whenever possible. Only use pesticides as a last resort, and if you do, be sure to wash fruits and vegetables thoroughly before consuming.

• **Eat a variety of foods** – We cannot predict what foods will be unintentionally contaminated by chemicals. The best defense against such a scenario is to eat a variety of foods, as previously discussed. This will limit the consumption of any one type of food with higher-than-normal concentrations of chemical contaminates.

• **Eat and store foods in containers designed for eating and drinking** – Do not store water and food in containers unless they are labelled as food grade. And don't reuse containers unless they are intended to be used for that purpose. For example, single-use water bottles and microwavable meal containers should be discarded after use. Remember that plastics are chemicals too.

• **Use household chemical products properly** – Most household products are deemed safe, however, if they are used improperly, exposure may increase to a level that is beyond safe limits. Examples of common household chemical products include paint, stains, cleaners, disinfectants, aerosol sprays, air fresheners, automobile fluids, mothballs, swimming pool chemicals, fabric conditioners, detergents, weed killers, and insect repellants. For all of these products, be sure to follow the instructions printed on the label for proper use, storage, and disposal. Do not use these products for anything other than their intended purpose and only use the recommended concentration.

Lifestyle Changes

Throughout this book, we have covered a number of ways to prevent dementia. To avoid sabotaging our efforts, we need to revisit a few risk factors detailed earlier in the book. Most people already know that smoking cigarettes is unhealthy. But, what about the risk factors that are not so obvious? The following are some additional suggestions to further reduce risk [48].

• **Deal with stress early** – Some stress can be beneficial in that it helps us overcome challenges. However, if stress is excessive and chronic, it can have long-term health ramifications and can also increase risk of dementia, as discussed earlier. Stress can be largely mitigated through exercise, sleep, and a healthy diet.

• **Get help for depression** – Depression, in and of itself, is a risk factor, but it can also lead to inactivity in other areas of life, compounding the risk of developing dementia. Consider getting medical treatment if you are experiencing symptoms.

• **Protect the head from severe or repeated injury** – Common sense measures include wearing a seat belt when driving and using a helmet when engaging in activities where the head is more vulnerable to injury. Examples of such activities include biking, skating, and contact sports.

• **Reduce brain exposure to cellphone radiation** – The easiest way to reduce exposure is to use a hands-free cellphone kit, or headset, when talking on a phone. These kits use Bluetooth technology, which emit less radiation than a typical cell phone, and will keep the higher power antenna away from the head. Alternatively, you can use the speakerphone feature to accomplish the same thing.

• **Take a break from using technological devices** – Try not to use and rely on smartphones and computers all the time. With the increased use of these devices, we forget to go outside, engage in physical activities, and interact with other people. Such technology is limiting our exposure to certain types of stimulus and this may increase our risk. Also, by relying on these devices for processing information, performing basic calculations, and remembering simple lists, we are using our brains less and less. As we already discussed, inactivity in certain areas of the brain can eventually lead to lack of function.

• **Check labels on over-the-counter and prescription medications** – Medications should be treated like potentially dangerous chemicals. They have side effects and, if misused, can be dangerous to long-term health, including brain health. Check the labels on all medications, even over-the-counter ones, to ensure you are using them properly. Do not use them for any other purpose other than what is intended. Check the expiration dates and if they are old, discard them.

Modern Treatments for Dementia

There are several prescribed drugs that treat symptoms of dementia (e.g. cholinesterase inhibitors, memantine). Such drugs can alleviate memory loss, confusion, and thinking and behavioral problems. There are also supervised non-drug therapies that are designed to help improve quality of life. These treatments may even be more beneficial if started early. Unfortunately, none of them can stop dementia from progressing or reverse the damage.

As far as prevention, there is no evidence that anything definitive can be done to prevent dementia in all individuals. However, every person is different. Even without such evidence, it does not mean that we cannot delay the onset of symptoms. What evidence we do have suggests that we can still control, to some extent, how the brain reorganizes and repairs itself, no matter how old we are or what condition we are in.

Advanced treatments for dementia such as gene therapies, vaccines, stem cell regeneration, and other forms of brain stimulation, are currently being researched [49]. However, even if they show promise, it is unlikely that they will be available in the short-term. After all, it takes years for such drugs and therapies to undergo tests and clinical trials before being released on the market.

The bottom line is that we cannot wait for a cure to take action.

Conclusion

There are a number of things we can do to prevent dementia and possibly reverse the effects. If we are already experiencing the early stages, we may be able to mitigate some of the symptoms and maintain a certain level of brain function to preserve quality of life. However, the most effective thing we can all do, right now, is take action to prevent it from occurring in the first place. It is important to start as early as possible.

To prevent dementia, we must avoid the risk factors that lead to dementia. We must also take action to make the brain more resilient to damage by engaging in a variety of brain stimulation activities. After reading this book, it should be clear how to accomplish this. The measures contained herein should be easy to start and convenient enough to keep up as we age.

By being proactive and improving brain health, we also improve overall health and reduce the risk of developing other chronic diseases. So, we have nothing to lose. One day, when modern medicine uncovers a cure for dementia, we will have more options. But, in the meantime, we have all the tools we need to fight back against dementia.

Bibliography

[1] Alzheimer's Association, "What is Dementia," [Online]. Available: http://www.alz.org/what-is-dementia.asp. [Accessed 31 October 2016].

[2] Center for Disease Control and Prevention, "Deaths and Mortality," U.S. Department of Health and Human Services, 7 October 2016. [Online]. Available: http://www.cdc.gov/nchs/fastats/deaths.htm.

[3] D. Goldschmidt, "Is Alzheimer's Disease Preventable?," CNN, 25 June 2015. [Online]. Available: http://www.cnn.com/2015/06/23/health/alzheimers-early-intervention/.

[4] National Institute on Aging, "The Changing Brain in Healthy Aging," U.S. Department of Health & Human Services, 22 January 2015. [Online]. Available: https://www.nia.nih.gov/alzheimers/publication/part-1-basics-healthy-brain/changing-brain-healthy-aging.

[5] Alzheimer's Association, "Types of Dementia," [Online]. Available: http://www.alz.org/dementia/types-of-dementia.asp. [Accessed 31 October 2016].

[6] National Stroke Association, "Vascular Dementia," [Online]. Available: http://www.stroke.org/we-can-help/survivors/stroke-recovery/post-stroke-conditions/cognition/vascular-dementia. [Accessed 31 October 2016].

[7] Mayfield Brain and Spine, "Anatomy of the Brain," University of Cincinnati Department of Neurosurgery, April 2016. [Online]. Available: http://www.mayfieldclinic.com/PE-AnatBrain.htm.

[8] J. Huang, "Brain Dysfunction by Location," Merck, [Online]. Available: http://www.merckmanuals.com/home/brain,-spinal-cord,-and-nerve-disorders/brain-dysfunction/brain-dysfunction-by-location. [Accessed 31 October 2016].

[9] World Health Organization, "Dementia," April 2016. [Online]. Available: http://www.who.int/mediacentre/factsheets/fs362/en/. [Accessed 31 October 2016].

[10] American Academy of Family Physicians, "Dementia Symptoms," April 2014. [Online]. Available: http://familydoctor.org/familydoctor/en/diseases-conditions/dementia/symptoms.html. [Accessed 31 October 2016].

[11] Alzheimer Society of Canada, "Risk Factors," 18 December 2014. [Online]. Available: http://www.alzheimer.ca/en/About-dementia/Alzheimer-s-disease/Risk-factors.

[12] National Institute on Aging, "Looking for the Causes of AD," U.S. Department of Health & Human Services, 22 January 2015. [Online]. Available: https://www.nia.nih.gov/alzheimers/publication/part-3-ad-research-better-questions-new-answers/looking-causes-ad.

[13] National Institutes of Health, "Health Topics," U.S. Department of Health and Human Services, [Online]. Available: https://www.nhlbi.nih.gov/health/health-topics/. [Accessed 31 October 2016].

[14] National Institutes of Health, "Causes of Diabetes," U.S. Department of Health and Human Services, August 2014. [Online]. Available: https://www.niddk.nih.gov/health-information/diabetes/causes.

[15] National Institutes of Health, "Alcohol Alert," U.S. Department of Health and Human Services, October 2004. [Online]. Available: http://pubs.niaaa.nih.gov/publications/aa63/aa63.htm.

[16] Alzheimer's Association, "Traumatic Brain Injury," Alzheimer's Association, [Online]. Available: http://www.alz.org/dementia/traumatic-brain-injury-head-trauma-symptoms.asp. [Accessed 31 October 2016].

[17] Y. Stern, "Cognitive reserve in ageing and Alzheimer's disease," *The Lancet Neurology*, vol. 11, no. 11, p. 1006–1012, November 2012.

[18] B. Tinker, "Common Over-the-counter Drugs Can Hurt Your Brain," CNN, 18 April 2016. [Online]. Available: http://www.cnn.com/2016/04/18/health/otc-anticholinergic-drugs-dementia/.

[19] The Fisher Center for Alzheimer's Research Foundation, "Air Pollution May Raise Dementia Risk," [Online]. Available: https://www.alzinfo.org/articles/air-pollution-raise-dementia-risk/. [Accessed 31 October 2016].

[20] N. Kounang, "Dangerous Chemicals are Hiding in Everyday Products," CNN, 1 July 2016. [Online]. Available: http://www.cnn.com/2016/07/01/health/everyday-chemicals-we-need-to-reduce-exposure-to/.

[21] L. O. Killin, J. M. Starr, I. J. Shiue and T. C. Russ, "Environmental risk factors for dementia: a systematic review," BMC Geriatrics, 12 October 2016. [Online]. Available: https://bmcgeriatr.biomedcentral.com/articles/10.1186/s12877-016-0342-y.

[22] U.S. News and World Report, "MIND Diet," U.S. News and World Report, [Online]. Available: http://health.usnews.com/best-diet/mind-diet. [Accessed 31 October 2016].

[23] United States Department of Agriculture, "2015-2020 Dietary Guidelines for Americans," United States Department of Agriculture, [Online]. Available: https://www.cnpp.usda.gov/2015-2020-dietary-guidelines-americans. [Accessed 31 October 2016].

[24] Cleveland Clinic, "Does the MIND Diet Boost Your Memory?," Cleveland Clinic, 31 August 2016. [Online]. Available: https://health.clevelandclinic.org/2016/08/mind-diet-boost-memory/.

[25] Medline Plus, "Drugs, Herbs, and Supplements," U.S. National Library of Medicine, [Online]. Available: https://medlineplus.gov/druginformation.html. [Accessed 31 October 2016].

[26] University of Maryland Medical Center, "Complementary and Alternative Medicine Guide," University of Maryland Medical Center, [Online]. Available: http://umm.edu/health/medical/altmed. [Accessed 31 October 2016].

[27] C. Balion, L. E. Griffith, L. Strifler, M. Henderson, C. Patterson, G. Heckman, D. J. Llewellyn and P. Raina, "Vitamin D, cognition, and dementia," *Neurology,* vol. 79(13), pp. 1397-1405, 2012.

[28] D. Kohn, "When Gut Bacteria Changes Brain Function," The Atlantic, 24 June 2015. [Online]. Available: http://www.theatlantic.com/health/archive/2015/06/gut-bacteria-on-the-brain/395918/.

[29] L. Sanders, "Microbes can Play Games with the Mind," Society for Science & the Public, 23 March 2016. [Online]. Available: https://www.sciencenews.org/article/microbes-can-play-games-mind.

[30] PennState Extension, "Prebiotics: How to Feed Your Good Bacteria," Penn State College of Agricultural Sciences, [Online]. Available: http://extension.psu.edu/health/functional-foods/health-nutrition-fact-sheets/prebiotics. [Accessed 31 October 2016].

[31] PennState Extension, "Probiotics: The Good Bugs," Penn State College of Agricultural Sciences, [Online]. Available: http://extension.psu.edu/health/functional-foods/health-nutrition-fact-sheets/probiotics-good-bugs. [Accessed 31 October 2016].

[32] G. Reynolds, "Walk, Jog or Dance: It's All Good for the Aging Brain," New York Times, 7 April 2016. [Online]. Available: http://well.blogs.nytimes.com/2016/04/07/sweat-smart/?_r=0.

[33] G. Reynolds, "Brain Benefits of Exercise Diminish After Short Rest," New York Times, 28 September 2016. [Online]. Available:

http://www.nytimes.com/2016/09/28/well/move/after-just-10-days-of-rest-brain-benefits-of-exercise-diminish.html?_r=0.

[34] Office of Disease Prevention and Health Promotion, "Physical Activity Guidelines for Americans," U.S. Department of Health and Human Services, [Online]. Available: https://health.gov/paguidelines/. [Accessed 31 October 2016].

[35] S. Liou, "Neurobiology," Huntington's Outreach Project for Education, at Stanford University, 26 June 2010. [Online]. Available: http://web.stanford.edu/group/hopes/cgi-bin/hopes_test/neuroplasticity/.

[36] S. Edwards, "Dancing and the Brain," Harvard Medical School, [Online]. Available: http://neuro.hms.harvard.edu/harvard-mahoney-neuroscience-institute/brain-newsletter/and-brain-series/dancing-and-brain. [Accessed 31 October 2016].

[37] M. Diament, "Friends Make you Smart," AARP, 21 November 2008. [Online]. Available: http://www.aarp.org/health/brain-health/info-11-2008/friends-are-good-for-your-brain.html.

[38] J. Carter, "Improving Brain Function with Exercise, Connectedness and Creativity," Parkinson's Disease Foundation, 2009. [Online]. Available: http://www.pdf.org/en/summer09_brain_function. [Accessed 31 October 2016].

[39] M. Healy, "Brain Training May Forestall Dementia Onset for Years, New Study Says," Los Angeles Times, 24 July 2016. [Online]. Available: http://www.latimes.com/science/sciencenow/la-sci-sn-brain-training-dementia-20160724-snap-story.html.

[40] CBS News, "Reminiscence Therapy helps trigger dementia patients' memories," CBS News, 19 November 2015. [Online]. Available: http://www.cbsnews.com/news/reminiscence-therapy-to-trigger-dementia-patients-memories/.

[41] J. Howard, "Do Brain Training Exercises Really Work?," CNN, 20 October 2016. [Online]. Available: http://www.cnn.com/2016/10/20/health/brain-training-exercises/.

[42] J. Hamilton, "Lack of Deep Sleep May Set the Stage for Alzheimer's," NPR, 4 January 2016. [Online]. Available: http://www.npr.org/sections/health-shots/2016/01/04/460620606/lack-of-deep-sleep-may-set-the-stage-for-alzheimers.

[43] Centers for Disease Control and Prevention, "Sleep and Chronic Disease," U.S. Department of Health and Human Services, 1 July 2013. [Online]. Available:

http://www.cdc.gov/sleep/about_sleep/chronic_disease.html.

[44] American Academy of Sleep Medicine, "Seven or more Hours of Sleep per Night: A Health Necessity for Adults," 1 June 2015. [Online]. Available: http://www.aasmnet.org/articles.aspx?id=5596.

[45] University of Maryland Medical Center, "Sleep Hygiene," [Online]. Available: http://ummidtown.org/programs/sleep/patients/sleep-hygiene. [Accessed 31 October 2016].

[46] National Health Service, "Pesticides and Dementia," 2 December 2010. [Online]. Available: http://www.nhs.uk/news/2010/12December/Pages/dementia-pesticide-use.aspx.

[47] Environmental Working Group, "EWG's 2016 Shopper's Guide to Pesticides in Produce," 2016. [Online]. Available: http://www.ewg.org/foodnews/summary.php. [Accessed 31 October 2016].

[48] Alzheimer's Association, "New Research Summary: Lifestyle Changes Help Reduce Risk of Cognitive Decline," 1 June 2015. [Online]. Available: http://www.alz.org/news_and_events_lifestyle_changes_help_reduce_risk.asp.

[49] National Health Service , "Is there a cure for dementia?," 17 June 2015. [Online]. Available: http://www.nhs.uk/Conditions/dementia-guide/Pages/dementia-cure.aspx.

www.ingramcontent.com/pod-product-compliance
Lightning Source LLC
Chambersburg PA
CBHW060642280326
41933CB00012B/2119